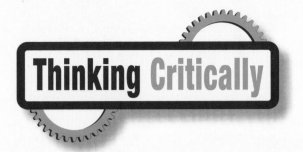

Thinking Critically: Biomedical Ethics

Andrea C. Nakaya

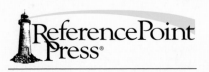

ReferencePoint
Press®

San Diego, CA

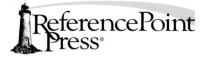

© 2015 ReferencePoint Press, Inc.
Printed in the United States

For more information, contact:
ReferencePoint Press, Inc.
PO Box 27779
San Diego, CA 92198
www. ReferencePointPress.com

Picture Credits:
AJ Photo/Science Source: 10
Steve Zmina: 16, 21, 29, 34, 41, 48, 55, 61

LIBRARY OF CONGRESS CATALOGING-IN-PUBLICATION DATA

Nakaya, Andrea C., 1976-
  Thinking critically : biomedical ethics / by Andrea C. Nakaya.
      pages cm. -- (Thinking critically)
  Audience: Grade 9 to 12.
  Includes bibliographical references and index.
  ISBN-13: 978-1-60152-674-8 (hardback)
  ISBN-10: 1-60152-674-1 (hardback)
  1. Medical ethics. 2. Bioethics. 3. Biomedical engineering. I. Title.
  R724.N347 2015
  174.2--dc23
                                                          2013047993

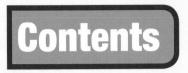
Contents

Foreword

"Literacy is the most basic currency of the knowledge economy we're living in today." Barack Obama (at the time a senator from Illinois) spoke these words during a 2005 speech before the American Library Association. One question raised by this statement is: What does it mean to be a literate person in the twenty-first century?

E.D. Hirsch Jr., author of *Cultural Literacy: What Every American Needs to Know*, answers the question this way: "To be culturally literate is to possess the basic information needed to thrive in the modern world. The breadth of the information is great, extending over the major domains of human activity from sports to science."

But literacy in the twenty-first century goes beyond the accumulation of knowledge gained through study and experience and expanded over time. Now more than ever literacy requires the ability to sift through and evaluate vast amounts of information and, as the authors of the Common Core State Standards state, to "demonstrate the cogent reasoning and use of evidence that is essential to both private deliberation and responsible citizenship in a democratic republic."

The Thinking Critically series challenges students to become discerning readers, to think independently, and to engage and develop their skills as critical thinkers. Through a narrative-driven, pro/con format, the series introduces students to the complex issues that dominate public discourse—topics such as gun control and violence, social networking, and medical marijuana. All chapters revolve around a single, pointed question such as Can Stronger Gun Control Measures Prevent Mass Shootings?, or Does Social Networking Benefit Society?, or Should Medical Marijuana Be Legalized? This inquiry-based approach introduces student researchers to core issues and concerns on a given topic. Each chapter includes one part that argues the affirmative and one part that argues the negative—all written by a single author. With the single-author format the predominant arguments for and against an issue can be synthesized into clear, accessible discussions supported by details and evidence including relevant facts, direct quotes, current examples, and statistical illustrations. All volumes include focus questions to guide students as they read each pro/con discussion, a list of key facts, and an annotated list of related organizations and websites for conducting further research.

The authors of the Common Core State Standards have set out the particular qualities that a literate person in the twenty-first century must have. These include the ability to think independently, establish a base of knowledge across a wide range of subjects, engage in open-minded but discerning reading and listening, know how to use and evaluate evidence, and appreciate and understand diverse perspectives. The new Thinking Critically series supports these goals by providing a solid introduction to the study of pro/con issues.

Biomedical Ethics

The Tuskegee syphilis experiment is one of the most infamous biomedical research studies ever conducted in the United States. It was done by the US Public Health Service between 1932 and 1972 and involved 399 African American men with the illness and 201 without. Syphilis is a sexually transmitted disease that can be treated effectively today, but in 1932 it was a major public health problem because doctors did not have a safe and effective way to treat it. Without treatment syphilis can lead to blindness, arthritis, brain damage, and death. The purpose of the study was to learn more about the effects of untreated syphilis on African American men. In order to monitor the natural progression of the disease, researchers purposely deceived the participants. They did not tell them they had syphilis or provide any form of treatment. By 1972 twenty-eight men had died of syphilis, one hundred others had died of related complications, at least forty wives had contracted it, and nineteen children had it from birth. Even when researchers learned in the 1940s that penicillin was a safe and effective treatment for syphilis, they withheld it from study participants.

Physician John C. Cutler, who was involved in the study, defended it as providing important scientific information for society. Cutler argued that the death of some was acceptable because the study had great benefits for society as a whole. "Some will die," he said in a 1993 documentary. "It's in the interest of the total society. These men in Tuskegee helped us learn how to treat syphilis among blacks. They were serving their race."[1] Although the study might have yielded some worthwhile information, few scientists today support such methods. A study that intentionally deceives and harms participants violates all standards of ethics.

Codes of Conduct

In order to protect society from unethical practices such as those that occurred in the Tuskegee experiment, the field of biomedical ethics has evolved. Bioethicists study the ethical issues that exist in relation to medicine and health care, try to decide what is right and wrong, and work to develop acceptable standards of conduct. Because medical technology is constantly changing, new ethical issues continue to arise, and bioethicists constantly face new questions. For example, science is bringing researchers closer to the point where it may be possible to clone a human being. But at the same time, ethicists wonder whether it will ever be ethical for researchers to create human life in this way. US president Barack Obama stresses that although technological advances are important, society must be vigilant about continually examining the resulting ethical issues. He says, "As our nation invests in science and innovation and pursues advances in biomedical research and health care, it's imperative that we do so in a responsible manner."[2]

To help ensure that medical professionals do consider ethical issues, various ethical codes of conduct exist. For example, the American Medical Association has established its Code of Medical Ethics, which provides ethical standards for a wide range of issues, such as physician-assisted suicide (PAS) and genetic testing. Bioethics advisers and commissions are also employed by research hospitals and universities to offer guidance about ethical issues. Even the US government has an ethics commission. The Presidential Commission for the Study of Bioethical Issues was created in 2009 to advise the government on issues ranging from human subjects research to genome sequencing.

Physician-Assisted Suicide

Even after extensive study by bioethicists, however, there is often no easy answer to biomedical ethics issues. For example, society is greatly divided over the ethics of PAS. PAS is when, at a patient's request, a physician provides a lethal dose of medicine that the patient can use to end his or her life. It is ethically controversial because it conflicts with the role of the doctor as healer. While some believe that sick people have the right to end their suffering, others insist that it is never ethical for a doctor to kill and that to do so will damage the doctor-patient relationship. Because it is so controversial, PAS is legally permitted in only a few places around the world. In the United States, the only states that allow it are Oregon, Montana, Washington, and Vermont. Assisted suicide is also legal in Belgium, Luxembourg, Netherlands, Switzerland, and Colombia.

Even where PAS is legal, however, it is not used very often. According to US public health records, for instance, seventy-seven people in Oregon and eighty-three people in Washington died through PAS in 2012. For Oregon, that was 0.2 percent of all deaths for 2012. In Washington, it represented a similarly small percentage of deaths. Nevertheless, the debate over allowing doctors to provide life-ending medicine to patients continues.

Genetic Testing

Another important topic in biomedical ethics is genetic testing. Genetic testing is continually becoming more advanced and more commonly used in the medical field. As a result, it continues to raise new questions about how much knowledge and control humans should have concerning their genetic makeup. One ethically controversial area of genetic testing is reproductive technology, where testing has become increasingly sophisticated. For example, doctors in fertility clinics routinely create and genetically test embryos before they implant them in the womb. Testing allows them to select embryos with or without certain characteristics. For example, many people use this technology to make sure they will not have a baby with certain genetic diseases and disabilities, such as cystic fibrosis or Down syndrome. Some people also use it to choose the sex of their baby. However, ethicists wonder whether manipulating genes is an appropriate use of the technology and whether these actions will have harmful consequences.

Another controversial type of testing is direct-to-consumer genetic testing, where consumers collect and send in their own DNA sample, then receive an analysis by mail, phone, or online. This type of testing is controversial because it does not necessarily involve a doctor or genetic counselor to help the consumer properly understand the results of the test. Ethicists worry that consumers may use this information without properly understanding it. In response to ethical concerns, direct-to-consumer testing service 23andMe announced in 2013 that it would temporarily stop providing testing information while undergoing review by the US Food and Drug Administration.

Embryonic Stem Cell Research

Embryonic stem cell research raises other questions involving biomedical ethics. Embryonic stem cells are found in a human embryo when it is just a few days old. These cells are pluripotent, which means they have the ability to grow into any type of cell in the body. Because of this ability, researchers believe that stem cells also have enormous potential for curing diseases, growing replacement organs and tissues, and illuminating understanding of human development.

Embryonic stem cells, usually about 150 of them, are taken from the embryo when it is about five days old. However, taking these cells causes the destruction of the embryo, and thus this research is highly controversial. Critics insist that an embryo is a human life, and regardless of the potential research benefits, it is always unethical to kill a human being. As a result of intense disagreement, embryonic stem cell research is subject to many restrictions in the United States and elsewhere.

Organ Donation

The field of organ donation is yet another example of how advances in medical technology have created ethical issues. Doctors now have the ability to transplant a number of organs—including lungs, hearts, kidneys, and livers—from donors to people whose own organs are failing. (Kidneys are the most commonly transplanted organ.) This technology saves many lives. However, the United States—like most other countries—has a huge shortage of available organs compared to what is needed. According to the US Department of Health and Human Services, in November

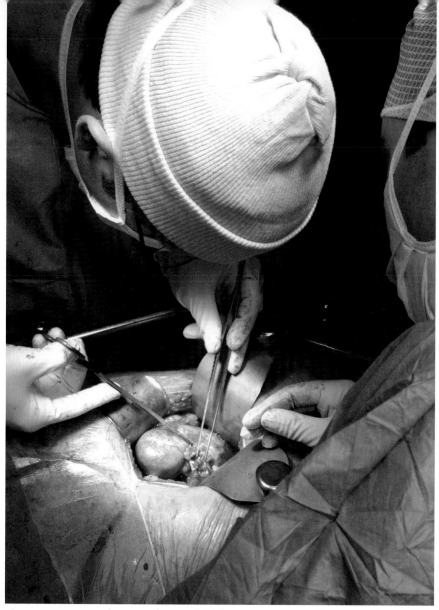

A surgeon transplants a donated kidney, giving an ill patient hope for new life. The limited supply of transplantable organs has created thorny ethical issues involving who should have priority for receiving these precious gifts of life.

2013 there were more than 120,000 people on the waiting list for organs. The department says that an average of eighteen people die each day because they do not receive the organs they need.

As a result of this scarcity of organs, there is disagreement over how they should be allocated. At present, the United States maintains a national registry of people who need organ transplants. Allocations are based on a number of criteria such as matching blood and tissue types, a consideration of how long the patient has been waiting, and the severity of his or her illness. Patients located closer to the available organ usually get higher priority, because once an organ is removed it only stays healthy for a short time. This system inevitably leads to ethical questions over who should have priority for obtaining organs and whether there are other ways to obtain organs without violating ethical standards. Because organs are scarce, any organ donation policy will result in some lives being saved and others lost.

Engaging in Medicine Responsibly

The field of medicine is an extremely powerful force in society. Medical professionals have the ability to dramatically change lives by transplanting organs, providing dying patients with lethal doses of medicine, or conducting genetic analysis. However, society must constantly be vigilant that such power is not abused. This is the role of biomedical ethics: to continually ask questions about what is right and wrong and about how society should decide what is ethical and what is not.

Chapter One

Should Physician-Assisted Suicide Be Legal?

Physician-Assisted Suicide Should Be Legal

- Terminally ill individuals should have the right to choose PAS.
- In some cases PAS is the best way for a doctor to help a patient.
- There is no evidence that PAS leads to abuses such as pressuring ill people to die.
- Legalization of PAS may actually reduce abuse.

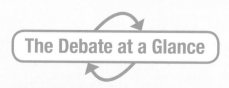

The Debate at a Glance

Physician-Assisted Suicide Should Not Be Legal

- Major medical organizations state that PAS is unethical.
- Helping a patient die is not compatible with the role of doctors.
- Rather than legalizing PAS, society needs to improve medical care.
- Legalizing PAS may lead to abuses such as pressuring ill people to die.

Physician-Assisted Suicide Should Be Legal

"I believe that people with a terminal illness have a right to die at a time and place of their own choosing."

—John M. Grohol is a doctor, author, and researcher.

John M. Grohol, "Death with Dignity: Why I Don't Want to Have to Starve Myself to Death," Psych Central, September 30, 2012. http://psychcentral.com.

Consider these questions as you read:

1. Do you agree with the argument that participating in PAS may be the best way for a physician to help a patient? Why or why not?
2. Can you think of an example where the right of one person to die might conflict with the rights of others? Explain.
3. How persuasive is the argument that legalizing PAS may reduce abuse? Which arguments provide the strongest support for this perspective, and why?

Editor's note: The discussion that follows presents common arguments made in support of this perspective, reinforced by facts, quotes, and examples taken from various sources.

Eight days before Canadian physician Donald Low died of brain cancer in 2013, he recorded a video that was posted on YouTube. In the video Low explains why he believes PAS should be legal. Low says he is not worried about dying. Rather, he worries about not having control over the way his life will end. He says, "I know it's going to end; it's never going to get better. So, I'm going to die, and what worries me is how I'm going to die."[3]

Low was frustrated by not having control over his own life and how it ended. He believed that PAS would have allowed him to die with dignity, but he did not have that option; PAS is not legal in Canada. So Low died a slow, painful death—something no one should be forced to do. Not everyone in this position would want to end their lives, but Low was not alone in his desire for a dignified end to his life. To those who made it impossible for him to achieve this end, he stated in his video: "I wish they could live in my body for 24 hours and I think they would change that opinion."[4]

The Right to Die with Dignity

Terminally ill people such as Low should have the right to choose PAS. These individuals are dying no matter what treatment their doctor provides, and they simply wish to have some control over how death occurs. It is unethical to deny them the means to a dignified death. Oregon resident Nora Miller talks about how her husband, Rick, chose PAS—which is legal in Oregon—after he was diagnosed with terminal lung cancer. She explains that PAS allowed him the dignified death that he wanted. She says, "The Oregon law allowed us to share his last moments and say our goodbyes while he was lucid and present, knowing he died on his own terms. My heart goes out to families who do not have this option, who must sit for hours or days or weeks as death takes their loved ones a centimeter at a time." In comparison, says Miller, her mother did not have the choice of PAS, and her death was very different; it was painful and undignified. She says, "My mother . . . [was] groggy from pain medication and hypoxia [when the body does not get enough oxygen], unable to recognize her own daughters at her bedside. My last memories of her are strongly colored by her pain and delirium."[5]

The Best Way to Help a Patient

While the traditional role of the doctor is to help patients stay healthy and treat them when they get sick, this does not mean that PAS is unethical. In some cases, such as terminal illness, it is appropriate for doctors to help suffering patients end their lives. David J. Mayo, board member of Death with Dignity, explains that the obligation of caring for patients includes helping those who are dying meet the end of life in a humane fashion—without fear and without suffering. He asks, "What possible good is served by denying escape from those final weeks of slow decline and suffering? And what horrible fear haunts many more terminal patients . . . terrified of how their final days might play out as circumstances strip them of every shred of control?"[6]

No matter how hard a doctor tries to relieve the pain and suffering of a patient, there will always be cases where relief is impossible. In these cases, when a patient asks for it, PAS may be the best choice. Timothy Quill, director of the Center for Ethics, Humanities and Palliative Care, argues that no matter how good medical care is, "a small percentage of dying patients will still experience suffering that can become intolerable and unacceptable." He says, "A subset of those will want assistance helping death come earlier rather than later."[7] Doctors are in the unique position of being able to ethically provide this help. In fact, to withhold assistance at this critical time in life would be far more unethical than the opposite.

> "What possible good is served by denying escape from those final weeks of slow decline and suffering?"[6]
>
> —David J. Mayo is a board member for the organization Death with Dignity.

No Evidence of Abuse

While critics charge that PAS is unethical because it leads to inadequate care or pressure on sick people to die, there is little evidence that abuse is occurring in places that have legalized the practice. Oregon legalized PAS in 1994 and Washington in 2008, and both states have numerous safeguards to prevent abuse. For example, PAS is only allowed for terminally ill patients with a life expectancy of six months or less, a second doctor must agree with the diagnosis, and the patient must request death twice verbally and at least once in writing. There is strong evidence that these safeguards are working. Before legalization, critics worried that vulnerable groups of people such as the elderly would feel pressure to end their lives because they lack end-of-life, or palliative, care.

No Evidence That Legalization Leads to Abuse

A common fear about legalization of PAS is that vulnerable groups of people such as the elderly, uneducated, or uninsured will be pressured into dying. However, data from Washington, where PAS is legal, shows little evidence to support this fear. Instead, this chart shows that the majority of Washington's PAS patients in 2011 and 2012 were terminal cancer patients, had medical insurance, had a high level of education, and were younger than seventy-five years old.

Characteristics of the Participants of the Death with Dignity Act Who Have Died	2011	2012
Age	%	%
18–44	3	1
45–54	10	2
55–64	23	30
65–74	29	33
75–84	20	23
85+	15	10
Education		
Less than high school	5	2
High school graduate	20	13
Some college	28	22
Baccalaureate or higher	46	48
Missing	1	1
Unknown (death certificate not received)		14
Underlying Illness		
Cancer	78	73
Neuro-degenerative disease (incl. ALS)	12	10
Respiratory disease (incl. COPD)	4	10
Heart disease	4	4
Other illnesses	2	3
Insurance Status		
Private only	34	22
Medicare or Medicaid only	40	55
Combination of private and Medicare/Medicaid	13	12
None	3	0
Unknown	10	11

Source: Washington State Department of Health, "Washington State Department of Health 2012 Death with Dignity Act Report: Executive Summary," 2013. www.doh.wa.gov.

Quill looks at data from Oregon and finds that these fears have not come true. He reports that overall, PAS only accounts for a small number of deaths every year, and these are generally not vulnerable groups of people. Instead, most people who choose to die this way are terminally ill cancer patients. In addition, most of the patients do not appear to be choosing PAS because of inadequate palliative care. What Quill found is that most of those who request help in dying have access to such care; 87.7 percent were enrolled in hospice.

Legalization May Reduce Abuse

Not only is there a lack of evidence that legalizing PAS leads to abuse, but legalization may actually reduce the likelihood of abuse. Even though PAS is illegal in most places, significant numbers of sick people do manage to end their lives anyway. For example, the organization Final Exit helps many sick people die by giving them information and guidance about suicide. Or family members sometimes help sick relatives die by giving them an overdose of medication. Such practices are widely reported. However, when this type of killing happens illegally, there is no regulation or oversight governing what occurs. In 2007 when Arizona resident Jana Van Voorhis decided she wanted to end her life, she contacted Final Exit. Two guides from the organization came to her house and instructed her in the use of a helium tank and hood to end her life. After she killed herself, the guides moved her body to make the death appear natural, and removed the helium tank and hood. The distressed family later said that Voorhis had been suffering from mental illness since her teens; they insisted that she needed medical help, not help in committing suicide. If not for Final Exit, they believe, Voorhis would still be alive.

> "A small percentage of dying patients will still experience suffering that can become intolerable and unacceptable."[7]
>
> —Timothy Quill is director of the Center for Ethics, Humanities and Palliative Care.

By legalizing a practice that is already occurring, the government can regulate it and prevent abuses—and eliminate the demand for organizations like Final Exit. The Netherlands Ministry of Foreign Affairs explains that this is one of the reasons that euthanasia (the act of ending the life of a person who is terminally ill) and PAS have been decriminalized in Netherlands. It maintains that these practices were already occurring before decriminalization and that the government changed the law because it did not want to ignore that fact. The ministry says, "The main aim of the policy is to bring matters into the open, to apply uniform criteria in assessing every case in which a doctor terminates life, and hence to ensure that maximum care is exercised in such exceptional cases."[8]

Physician-assisted suicide should be available as an end-of-life option under specific circumstances for those who want it. Helping terminally ill patients end their lives is compatible with the role of the doctor. Death is a part of life, and doctors have an ethical responsibility to assist their patients when needed in this final stage of life. Only by legalizing physician-assisted suicide will such care be possible.

Physician-Assisted Suicide Should Not Be Legal

"The College does not support legalization of physician-assisted suicide. . . . The practice might undermine patient trust; distract from reform in end-of-life care; and be used in vulnerable patients."

—The American College of Physicians is a national internal medicine organization.

American College of Physicians, *Ethics Manual,* 6th ed., 2013. www.acponline.org.

Consider these questions as you read:

1. Do you think that helping a patient die can ever be compatible with the role of a doctor? Why or why not?
2. How persuasive is the argument that society could eliminate the need for PAS by improving patient care? Explain.
3. Taking into account the facts and ideas presented in this discussion, how persuasive is the argument that PAS should not be legal? Which facts and ideas are strongest, and why?

Editor's note: The discussion that follows presents common arguments made in support of this perspective, reinforced by facts, quotes, and examples taken from various sources.

Many attempts to legalize PAS have been made in the United States. Oregon and Washington succeeded through ballot initiatives where citizens voted on the issue, Vermont by passing a legislative bill, and Montana through a decision by that state's supreme court. Similar efforts in other states have failed. According to the Patients Rights Council, since January 1994 lawmakers in twenty-seven states have introduced 135 bills aimed at giving legal status to PAS. Only in Vermont has physician-assisted suicide been made legal through legislative action. Legislators do not operate within a vacuum; these results suggest that they lacked support from their constituents for the idea of allowing doctors to give their patients the means to kill themselves when requested. The lesson here is that most Americans recognize that it is unethical for a physician to participate in intentionally ending the life of a patient and do not support the legalization of this practice.

Not Compatible with the Role of Doctor

Numerous professional medical associations strongly oppose PAS because they believe it is unethical. For example, the World Medical Association urges physicians to refrain from participating in this practice and states that it should be condemned by the medical professions. The American Medical Association also advises against it. It says, "Allowing physicians to participate in assisted suicide would cause more harm than good." Additionally, it warns, "Physician-assisted suicide is fundamentally incompatible with the physician's role as healer, would be difficult or impossible to control, and would pose serious societal risks."[9] PAS is simply not compatible with the role of a doctor. Eric Wasylenko, a Canadian physician who specializes in palliative care, explains that it is never right for physicians to intentionally kill patients. He says, "It is not within the role of the physician or the practice of medicine to actually deliberately cause someone's death, even if they've asked for it." Instead, he says, "the role of physicians and medical care is to support people in their life until their natural death, not to kill them artificially or in advance of their natural death."[10]

> "It is not within the role of the physician or the practice of medicine to actually deliberately cause someone's death, even if they've asked for it."[10]
>
> —Eric Wasylenko is a Canadian physician who specializes in palliative care.

Medical practitioner David Blazer worries that giving anyone the power to kill, even a doctor, will inevitably lead to problems. For example, he says, "there will be those physicians who find it too easy, who find it in vogue, who confront the issue with too little consideration of

Legalization May Lead to Abuse

In physician-assisted suicide, a doctor provides a patient with a prescription for lethal medication. The patient then takes this medication at a time of his or her choosing, sometimes without the prescribing doctor or other medical professional present. This lack of medical supervision means that there is a real potential for abuse. For example, sick people might be pressured to die by family so that they are not a burden. Data from Oregon, where PAS is legal, shows that overall there may be a significant lack of medical supervision when patients die through PAS. This chart shows deaths in Oregon under the state's Death with Dignity Act. It reveals that in many cases, either no health care provider was present at the time the lethal dose was taken or no information was available to indicate whether a health care provider was present.

Health-Care Provider Present	1998–2011	2012	Total
When medication was ingested			
• Prescribing physician	100	8	108
• Other provider, prescribing physician not present	231	4	235
• No provider	72	1	73
• Unknown	123	64	187
At time of death			
• Prescribing physician	89 (17%)	7 (9%)	96 (16%)
• Other provider, prescribing physician not present	254 (49%)	4 (5%)	258 (44%)
• No provider	171 (33%)	66 (86%)	237 (40%)
• Unknown	12	0	12

Source: Oregon Public Health Division, "Oregon's Death with Dignity Act—2012," 2013. http://public.health.oregon.gov.

options or ramifications." In his opinion, "It is too dangerous a license to give to anyone: the license to end a life."[11]

Provide Adequate Care for Dying Patients

Rather than participating in PAS, physicians should focus on making patients as comfortable as possible at the end of their lives. The American

Medical Association explains that there are many ways to alleviate suffering without resorting to killing the patient. It says, "Instead of participating in assisted suicide, physicians must aggressively respond to the needs of patients at the end of life." It explains the importance of good palliative care: "Multidisciplinary interventions should be sought including specialty consultation, hospice care, pastoral support, family counseling, and other modalities. Patients near the end of life must continue to receive emotional support, comfort care, adequate pain control, respect for patient autonomy, and good communication."[12] The real problem is not that doctors cannot legally help their patients commit suicide; it is that too many dying patients do not receive good end-of-life care. This is the problem that society must address so that sick and dying patients do not see suicide as the only means of relief. Numerous studies show that many terminally ill people do not receive sufficient palliative care. For example, in a 2011 report the Center to Advance Palliative Care and the National Palliative Care Research Center state that millions of Americans do not have access to palliative care when they need it. The report says, "Where there is approximately one cardiologist for every 71 persons experiencing a heart attack and one oncologist for every 141 newly diagnosed cancer patients, there is only one palliative medicine physician for every 1,200 persons living with a serious or life-threatening illness."[13]

It is understandable that terminally ill people who are experiencing pain, depression, and fear might wish for death. It is also well known that when patients in this state receive appropriate care, they no longer seek a way to prematurely end their lives. Mary E. Harned, staff counsel for Americans United for Life, explains, "Studies have revealed that when offered personal support and palliative care, most patients adapt and continue in ways they might not have anticipated."[14]

The Very Real Dangers of Legalization

When PAS is a legal option, however, sick people may not have the opportunity to find ways to adapt and continue because they may choose to die instead. Doctor Kenneth Stevens argues that the availability of assisted suicide may cause patients to give up too quickly. To support this view, he offers the example of Oregon resident Jeanette Hall, who was diagnosed with cancer in 2000 and told that she had six months to live. Hall came to Stevens to request PAS; however, he refused and inspired her to fight the disease instead. As a result, Hall ended up beating the cancer and was alive more than ten years later. Stevens believes that in Hall's case, the legality of PAS was dangerous because it almost led her to end her life prematurely. He says, "The mere presence of legal assisted suicide steered her to suicide."[15] In addition to influencing patients to give up too soon, the legalization of PAS could easily lead to abuses, especially involving vulnerable populations of elderly and disabled people. By legalizing physician-assisted suicide, society suggests that not all lives have value, thereby endangering the most vulnerable among us. Patrick Lee, who is John N. and Jamie D. McAleer Chair in Bioethics at Franciscan University of Steubenville in Ohio, explains that it is important for society to protect life no matter what the circumstances, and this means never allowing PAS. He says, "If a culture regards human life as inviolable, that fact protects all of us; if not, then the most vulnerable among us—especially the elderly and the disabled—are in danger." He explains, "If the law against PAS were rescinded and PAS were widely practiced, that would send the message that in many cases a person's life is simply not worth living."[16] The effect of such a message could have devastating consequences for those who are most vulnerable.

Evidence of abuse can be found in countries that allow PAS. Researcher José Pereira has reviewed international data on legalized euthanasia and PAS. Despite attempts to institute safeguards to prevent abuse, he has found widespread evidence that the safeguards are not working. For example, he says, large numbers of cases in Belgium and Netherlands are not reported to authorities, which means they are not reviewed to see whether the law was properly followed. He also says that requirements for consultation with a second physician are widely ignored. Overall, he says, "there is evidence . . . that safeguards are ineffective and

> "If the law against PAS were rescinded and PAS were widely practiced, that would send the message that in many cases a person's life is simply not worth living."[16]
>
> —Patrick Lee is John N. and Jamie D. McAleer Chair in Bioethics at Franciscan University of Steubenville.

that many people who should not be euthanized or receive PAS are dying by those means."[17]

The legalization of physician-assisted suicide is not the way to help dying people find peace in their final days. It is an unethical use of those schooled in the skills of healing and medicine. The only ethical way to help dying people cope with illness, pain, and death is for society to make an absolute commitment to provide high-quality palliative care.

Chapter Two

Should Society Allow Genetic Testing?

Genetic Testing Offers Many Benefits

- Testing can help doctors provide more effective treatments.
- Genetic testing makes it easier to prevent health problems.
- Direct-to-consumer testing helps more people access their genetic information.
- Prenatal genetic testing helps parents prepare for special-needs babies.

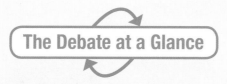

The Debate at a Glance

Genetic Testing Poses Many Problems

- The reduction of genetic diseases through prenatal testing is harmful to society.
- Knowing the results of a genetic test negatively impacts some people.
- Genetic testing can result in discrimination.
- Direct-to-consumer testing can mislead or misinform consumers.

Genetic Testing Offers Many Benefits

"For the first time ever, [because of genetic testing] we are looking at the chance to cure major diseases, possibly before they take hold. . . . We are living on the edge of a brave new world where the possibility of living without the health problems that have plagued us for generations is within sight."

—Emma G. Keller is a journalist.

Emma G. Keller, "Should We Fear DNA Testing?," *Guardian* (Manchester, UK), November 3, 2013. www .theguardian.com.

Consider these questions as you read:

1. How strong is the argument that genetic testing can dramatically improve health care? Explain your answer.
2. Do you agree that direct-to-consumer testing is a valuable tool for consumers? Why or why not?
3. Which pieces of evidence in this discussion provide the strongest support for the view that genetic testing offers many benefits? Why do you think they are the strongest?

Editor's note: The discussion that follows presents common arguments made in support of this perspective, reinforced by facts, quotes, and examples taken from various sources.

Warfarin is a commonly prescribed drug for patients who are at risk for heart attacks, strokes, and blood clots. It thins the blood, thus making these health problems less likely. However, although this drug can be very effective, it can also cause internal bleeding and death if the patient takes a dose that is too high. The problem is that the right dose varies by patient, and doctors often have trouble determining exactly what it should be. As the doctor experiments with various doses, there is a risk that the patient might die from either too little or too much warfarin.

Genetic testing offers a potential solution to this problem because researchers have discovered that genetic variations in individual patients can affect how the body interacts with warfarin. According to authors Lee Gutkind and Pagan Kennedy, "Studies indicate that integrating genetic testing with warfarin therapy—that is, screening patients before prescribing an initial dose of the drug—could prevent as many as 85,000 serious bleeding events and 17,000 strokes annually."[18] This is only one example of the benefits of genetic testing. Testing gives doctors vital information that allows them to better understand how to treat patients and improve health. It has the potential to save millions of lives and to dramatically improve health care—and not using this tool would be unethical.

Improving Health Care

Genetic testing can greatly improve health care. As the warfarin example reveals, it can do this by making personalized medicine possible. With personalized medicine, treatment strategies are based on genetic analysis of each patient, rather than on standard recommendations for a particular illness or drug. This type of treatment offers great promise. Paul Ravetto works at Qiagen, a company involved with molecular biology technology. He explains, "Through testing for specific genetic variations related to certain biomarkers, health professionals can choose from different treatment options to achieve the best possible therapeutic results and avoid unnecessary treatments."[19]

Additionally, genetic testing can provide information on the likelihood of a person's developing certain diseases. This could allow doctors to make early diagnoses and begin preventive measures before a condition surfaces or worsens. By working on prevention rather than treatment, both money and lives can be saved. At present, without genetic testing many illnesses are not discovered until they have already inflicted serious damage on a person's body. Gutkind and Kennedy give the example of pancreatic cancer, the fourth leading cause of death from cancer in the United States. They say, "Pancreatic cancer is a silent enemy; it grows secretly, undetectable, for decades. When it is discovered it is almost always too late to take action: pancreatic cancer is usually discovered only after it has spread to other organs." They report, "Fewer than 5% of those diagnosed with pancreatic cancer are alive five years later."[20] Being able to catch this cancer earlier through genetic testing could save many lives.

In 2013 actress Angelina Jolie underwent genetic testing to determine her risk for cancer. Jolie has a family history of cancer; among others, her mother died from ovarian cancer, and her aunt died from breast cancer. Genetic testing revealed that Jolie had a mutation of the BRCA1 gene, which greatly increases the chance of developing both breast and ovarian cancer. She says, "My doctors estimated that I had an 87 percent risk of breast cancer and a 50 percent risk of ovarian cancer." Because Jolie was able to obtain this genetic information, she could take action to protect her health. She chose to undergo a preventive double mastectomy, a procedure that entails removing both breasts. She says that following the surgery, "my chances of developing breast cancer have dropped from 87 percent to under 5 percent. I can tell my children that they don't need to fear they will lose me to breast cancer."[21]

> "Through testing for specific genetic variations related to certain biomarkers, health professionals can choose from different treatment options to achieve the best possible therapeutic results and avoid unnecessary treatments."[19]
>
> —Paul Ravetto works at Qiagen, a company involved with molecular biology technology.

Direct-to-Consumer Genetic Testing

The development of direct-to-consumer genetic testing has made it even easier for people to obtain information about their genes and, if needed, take steps to improve their health or prevent illness. With direct-to-consumer testing, customers order a testing kit and submit a DNA sample, such as saliva, by mail for testing. Such tests do not require a visit to a doctor or a lab. When the test is complete, the individual can view the results online. Jill Uchiyama underwent this type

Caregivers See Value in Genetic Screening for Fragile X Syndrome

Genetic testing can detect many health conditions, and research shows that many people believe such testing and detection is beneficial. Fragile X syndrome is a genetic condition that causes a range of developmental problems including learning disabilities and cognitive impairment. This graph shows the results of a study of 1,099 caregivers of children with this syndrome. Researchers asked their opinions about genetic testing for fragile X syndrome before and during pregnancy, in newborns, and in children who show possible signs of the syndrome. Overall, researchers found that most respondents either agreed or strongly agreed that free, voluntary genetic screening should be offered in all of these situations.

Percentage of Caregivers Who Agree That Free, Voluntary Genetic Testing Should Be Offered at Different Times

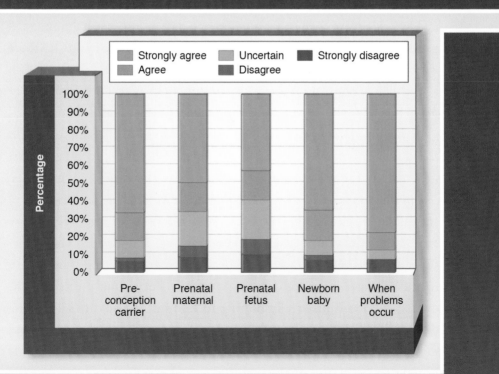

Source: Donald B. Bailey Jr., Ellen Bishop, Melissa Raspa, and Debra Skinner, "Caregiver Opinions About Fragile X Population Screening," *Genetics in Medicine*, 2012. www.nature.com.

of testing. She says that her test revealed some interesting facts but also some helpful health information. Says Uchiyama:

> I got to learn what traits I have such as difficulty with metabolizing caffeine, the sprinter gene [a gene that allows a person to produce explosive bursts of speed], and a tendency toward sneezing in sunlight along with dozens of other traits. I got to see what diseases and conditions I have a predisposition toward and ones that I have less of a disposition toward. That helped me tremendously in putting my attention on particular pieces of my health and raising my awareness on preventative measures.[22]

Research shows that most people have a strong desire to learn about potential health problems and take action before they arise. Direct-to-consumer testing helps them do this, and because it is generally easier and less expensive than other types of genetic testing, it is helping to expand access to genetic knowledge to almost anyone who wants it. There is no ethical reason to keep people from obtaining more information about themselves. And if direct-to-consumer testing encourages them to make healthier choices, that is even better.

Knowing about potential problems early and being able to act on that knowledge are the primary reasons people undergo genetic testing. This is the conclusion of a study published in 2013 in in the *Journal of Community Genetics*. In that study Katherine Wasson and colleagues evaluated the responses and reactions of twenty primary care patients who underwent genetic testing. They state: "Many participants repeatedly articulated a desire to gain knowledge and act on it as a key motivation for deciding to test."[23] For example, one respondent said, "I was just really hoping to find out if I am at risk for any diseases that run in my family. . . . My grandmother had diabetes and my mother had heart problems, my father had cancer, and I was just hoping to see if any of these things, you know, if I had any genetic strain of these types of diseases."[24]

Prenatal Genetic Testing

Another beneficial use of genetic testing is in the field of reproductive medicine. It is commonly used to screen embryos and fetuses for abnormalities such as Down syndrome. Having this information allows a couple to make an informed decision about whether or not to have a baby with such a condition. If they choose to continue with the pregnancy and the baby is born with a serious genetic abnormality, they will have had time to prepare themselves for the unique challenges that baby will bring. In an online forum about whether or not prenatal testing is a good idea, a number of parents state that they are grateful for the knowledge genetic testing gave them. One respondent says, "I would rather have a heads up than be blindsided and unprepared."[25] Another says, "I'm glad I did get it done 'cause now I'm more prepared to handle a special needs child."[26]

> "[Testing] helped me tremendously in putting my attention on particular pieces of my health and raising my awareness on preventative measures."[22]
>
> —Jill Uchiyama underwent genetic testing through the company 23andMe.

Genetic testing is not a panacea, but it is an important tool. It can provide doctors and patients with critical information and allow them to make informed decisions and, when called for, to take preventive action. To deny people the use of such an important and beneficial tool would be unethical.

Genetic Testing Poses Many Problems

"The practice of genetic testing and screening has created moral controversies about who should be tested and what should be done with the results."

—The University of Missouri School of Medicine, Columbia, Missouri.

University of Missouri School of Medicine, "Genetic Testing and Screening," June 8, 2011. http://ethics .missouri.edu.

Consider these questions as you read:

1. Do you think society will be harmed by the decreasing number of children born with disabilities such as Down syndrome? Why or why not?

2. How strong is the argument that genetic testing may lead to discrimination? Explain your answer.

3. Do you agree that direct-to-consumer genetic testing might be harmful because consumers might misunderstand their testing results? Why or why not?

Editor's note: The discussion that follows presents common arguments made in support of this perspective, reinforced by facts, quotes, and examples taken from various sources.

In a 2012 article in *Slate*, writer and filmmaker Jasmeet Sidhu writes about a Canadian woman whom she calls Megan Simpson (not her real name). Simpson always wished for a daughter to share her interests of sewing, baking, and doing hair. However, her first two children were boys. Trying a third time, Simpson was devastated to find out that she was pregnant with yet another boy. She says, "I lay in bed and cried for weeks."[27] Desperate for a girl, she turned to genetic testing. Fertility doctors are able to use genetic testing to test the sex of embryos before they are implanted, thus allowing selection of either a boy or girl. After two attempts to create and implant a viable female embryo, Simpson finally had her baby girl. She says, "My husband and I stared at our daughter for that first year. She was worth every cent."[28] Genetic testing can bring great happiness while at the same time posing many ethical problems.

In cases of sex selection, ethicists worry about the implications of spending so much time and money to ensure that a child is a certain sex. Sidhu reports that Simpson's girl took nearly four years and $40,000. While the couple was clearly happy with the child, what happens when a child specifically selected—and paid for—does not turn out to be the person the parents envisioned? The potential harms of such a situation, to both parents and the child, are innumerable.

Prenatal Testing and Disabilities

Although the Simpsons used genetic testing for sex selection, it can also be used to detect abnormalities such as Down syndrome or spina bifida in the fetus. Having this information before birth allows people to make decisions about continuing the pregnancy or undergoing an abortion. Research shows that the number of babies born with these disabilities is decreasing, thanks in large part to prenatal genetic testing. Some ethicists believe this sends the wrong message to people with disabilities: It suggests they are somehow inferior and not worthy of life.

In fact, society benefits immensely from the variety of people who make up any given community, including those with genetic disabilities. Researchers Daniel Allott and Neumary George state, "There's growing evidence that people with disabilities provide something unique and meaningful to those they encounter. Numerous studies have shown that children with disabilities help cultivate the virtues of kindness, patience, and empathy in family members and friends."[29] Courtney and Trafford Kane of Swansea, Massachusetts, have a daughter with Down syndrome. When prenatal testing revealed her condition, the Kanes decided not to have an abortion—and they have never regretted their decision. The *Boston Globe* reports, "The Kanes say they are part of a club that no one would think they want to join, but that they would never want to leave."[30]

Prenatal Testing Increases Down Syndrome Abortions

Genetic testing can determine whether a baby is likely to be born with Down syndrome, and a positive test leads many prospective parents to abort the fetus. This sends the strong message that people born with Down syndrome are not worthy of life. For this reason, genetic testing is neither ethical nor beneficial. This chart summarizes the results of nine hospital-based studies on Down syndrome testing and abortion rates. It reveals that an average of 85.4 percent of people in these studies chose to terminate the pregnancy after learning that their baby would likely be born with Down syndrome.

Author (Year)	State	Institution	Study years	Pregnancies with Down syndrome by prenatal diagnosis (number)	Termination following prenatal diagnosis of Down syndrome	
					number	percent
Shaffer (2006)	CA	University of California at San Francisco	1983–2003	449	391	87.1%
Benn (1998)	CT	University of Connecticut	1992–1996	27	23	85.2%
Wray (2007)	DC	Georgetown University Hospital	2002–2004	10	6	60.0%
Caruso (1998)	MA	Brigham and Women's Hospital	1972–1974 1979–1994	31	27	87.1%
Brit (2000)	MI	Wayne State University	1989–1998	144	129	89.6%
Kramer (1998)	MI	Wayne State University	1989–1997	145	126	86.9%
Pemi (2006)	NY	New York Weill-Cornell Medical Center	2003–2004	22	19	86.4%
Perry (2007)	NY	University of Rochester Strong Memorial Hospital	1997–2005	59	43	72.9%
Horger (2001)	SC	University of South Carolina	1972–2000	37	25	67.6%
Average				924	789	85.4%

Source: Jamie L. Natoli et al., "Prenatal Diagnosis of Down Syndrome: A Systematic Review of Termination Rates," *Prenatal Diagnosis*, February 2012. http://onlinelibrary.wiley.com.

Testing for Disease Risk

Genetic testing raises a host of ethical issues—and not just involving births. More and more genetic testing is being used to determine a person's risk for developing certain illnesses. For example, genetic testing can be used to determine the risk of breast cancer in women who have a mutation in either of two genes known as BRCA1 and BRCA2. A positive test for the mutated BRCA gene does not mean that a woman will develop cancer. It means that she has a greatly increased chance of developing breast cancer or ovarian cancer. The problem is that many people do not properly understand the uses and implications of genetic tests such as this. As a result, some patients might undergo unnecessary tests, receive poorly interpreted results, or miss out on tests that could be beneficial. All of these possibilities can impact patient health.

In recent years a significant number of women with a higher genetic risk for breast cancer have chosen to undergo double mastectomies to lower that risk. However, research suggests that some might not fully understand the implications of genetic results and might be rushing into surgery that is also risky. A double mastectomy and reconstructive breast surgery is a major ordeal with life-changing consequences, and the fact is that if a woman does develop breast cancer, she actually has a high chance of survival. According to a 2013 NBC News report, when it is caught in the earliest stages, the survival rate for breast cancer is 93 percent. Some ethicists wonder whether some of the women undergoing double mastectomies are doing so because they are overestimating their risk of dying from breast cancer based on the results of inconclusive genetic tests.

A further ethical problem exists when genetic testing is done for illnesses that cannot be prevented or cured. An example of such a case is testing for Huntington's disease, a neurological condition that starts between ages thirty and fifty. Patients with Huntington's slowly lose muscle

> "There's growing evidence that people with disabilities provide something unique and meaningful to those they encounter."[29]
>
> —Daniel Allott and Neumary George are writers.

and brain function and eventually die. Even though it is possible to do a genetic test to identify whether or not a person will develop Huntington's, there is no way to prevent the development of the disease or to cure it. Writer Bruce Grierson argues that in the case of Huntington's, genetic testing is not beneficial. He says, "For most people a Huntington's diagnosis is toxic knowledge—a piece of news that clouds rather than clarifies. . . . Knowledge of the disease . . . shades every day on earth thereafter with new problems and impossible decisions, and absolutely nothing can be done about the underlying condition."[31]

Potential for Discrimination

Genetic testing that reveals conditions such as Huntington's is also unethical because it has the potential to lead to discrimination against people based on their genetics. Although the government has passed certain legislation to prevent discrimination, such as the Genetic Information Nondiscrimination Act, this legislation does not cover all circumstances. For example, the act prohibits discrimination by health insurance companies but does not address companies that sell life insurance, disability insurance, or long-term-care insurance.

One example of the potential for discrimination is in people who undergo genetic testing to determine their likelihood of developing Alzheimer's disease. This disease gradually takes away a person's memory and other intellectual capabilities; those who develop it often end up needing care in a nursing home or assisted-living facility. Such care would be covered by long-term-care insurance, and so people who find out they have a higher chance of developing Alzheimer's often purchase this type of insurance. However, insurance companies that provide long-term-care coverage are not prohibited from looking at test results and using that information to save money by refusing to insure people who are likely to develop Alzheimer's or charging them higher rates.

Direct-to-Consumer Genetic Testing

Rather than undergoing genetic testing through their doctor, some people choose direct-to-consumer genetic testing. However, this type of testing is problematic because it has a high potential for being misunderstood. The National Institutes of Health (NIH) explains that health risks cannot be predicted on the basis of test results alone. It says, "Genetic testing provides only one piece of information about a person's health—other genetic and environmental factors, lifestyle choices, and family medical history also affect a person's risk of developing many disorders."[32] In order to properly understand the way all these factors work together, the average person needs the help of a genetic counselor when reviewing test results; however, in direct-to-consumer testing there is often no such help. The NIH warns, "Without guidance from a healthcare provider, they may make important decisions about treatment or prevention based on inaccurate, incomplete, or misunderstood information about their health."[33]

> "Genetic testing provides only one piece of information about a person's health— other genetic and environmental factors, lifestyle choices, and family medical history also affect a person's risk of developing many disorders."[32]
>
> —The NIH conducts medical research in order to improve the health of Americans.

Genetic testing can result in discrimination against people with disabilities or in discrimination based on other information revealed by test results. It can also be problematic when people do not fully understand the results or when they discover a problem in their genetics that they are powerless to fix. Overall, genetic testing causes many ethical problems.

Chapter Three

Is Embryonic Stem Cell Research Ethical?

Embryonic Stem Cell Research Is Ethical

- The potential benefits justify embryonic stem cell research.
- Destruction of the early embryo is ethical because it is not a real person.
- It is ethical to use excess embryos from fertility clinics for research.
- The government should provide funding for embryonic stem cell research.

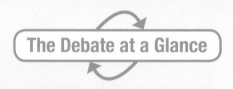

The Debate at a Glance

Embryonic Stem Cell Research Is Not Ethical

- It is morally wrong to destroy an embryo, regardless of the potential benefits.
- There are other, ethical alternatives to embryonic stem cell research.
- It is unethical to use surplus embryos from fertility clinics for research.
- The government should not provide funding for embryonic stem cell research.

Embryonic Stem Cell Research Is Ethical

"Human embryonic stem-cell research is not only ethical, it is an essential field to pursue to make key advances in biomedical research."

—Dan S. Kaufman is associate director at the University of Minnesota Stem Cell Institute.

Dan S. Kaufman, comment on *The Survival Doctor* (blog), "Embryonic Stem-Cell Research: Experts Debate Pros and Cons," February 14, 2013. www.thesurvivaldoctor.com.

Consider these questions as you read:

1. Do you agree with the argument that embryonic stem cell research should be pursued because of its enormous potential? Why or why not?
2. Do you agree that it is ethical to use excess embryos from fertility clinics for stem cell research? Why or why not?
3. Taking into account the facts and arguments presented in this discussion, how persuasive is the argument that embryonic stem cell research is ethical? Which piece of evidence is the weakest, and which is the strongest?

Editor's note: The discussion that follows presents common arguments made in support of this perspective, reinforced by facts, quotes, and examples taken from various sources.

Because embryonic stem cells have the ability to change into any kind of cell in the body, researchers believe they hold enormous potential for treating many kinds of illnesses. One research goal involving these cells is to create replacement tissues to transplant into sick patients; for example, a new heart for a person whose heart is failing. However, the human body is very likely to reject cells that are not a genetic match, so the first goal of researchers is to create embryonic stem cells that are a genetic match for individual patients. In 2013 a group of researchers led by Shoukhrat Mitalipov announced that they had successfully done this. They reported that they had used a human egg from a volunteer, then inserted DNA from a human skin cell. Finally, they stimulated the egg to develop into an embryo. They showed that this embryo could produce healthy stem cells with the same genes as the skin cell, thus providing a genetic match with the person who provided the skin cells. Researchers believe this is an important step toward being able to grow replacement tissues or organs that are specifically matched to patients. If researchers can do this, they could alleviate the suffering of millions of people. Taking stem cells from an embryo results in the destruction of the embryo; however, the enormous potential demonstrated by Mitalipov's and others' research proves embryonic stem cell research to be ethical.

Enormous Potential

In addition to being able to create replacement organs and tissue, researchers believe, embryonic stem cells also have the potential to cure many different diseases. The Americans for Cures Foundation says, "Stem cell research is perhaps the most exciting medical technology of the 21st Century. Stem cells hold the promise of treatments and cures for more than 70 major diseases and conditions that affect millions of people, including diabetes, Parkinson's, Alzheimer's, cancer, multiple sclerosis, Lou Gehrig's Disease (ALS), spinal cord injuries, blindness, and HIV/AIDS."[34]

> "Stem cell research is perhaps the most exciting medical technology of the 21st Century."[34]
>
> —The Americans for Cures Foundation, an organization formed to advance the field of stem cell research and regenerative medicine.

The potential to alleviate so much human suffering makes embryonic stem cell research ethical. In fact, as executive director of the Alliance for Aging Research Daniel Perry says, "Embryonic stem cells have a virtually unlimited future. . . . It would be truly immoral if the nation *does not* move to capitalize on the tantalizing potential of these new medical treatments to improve the lives of millions of people suffering from devastating and life-threatening diseases."[35]

Most Americans Believe Embryonic Stem Cell Research Is Ethical

Between 2003 and 2013, Gallup polled Americans about whether they believed embryonic stem cell research was morally acceptable. This graph shows the results and reveals that over that period of time, a majority of Americans consistently agreed that this research is morally acceptable.

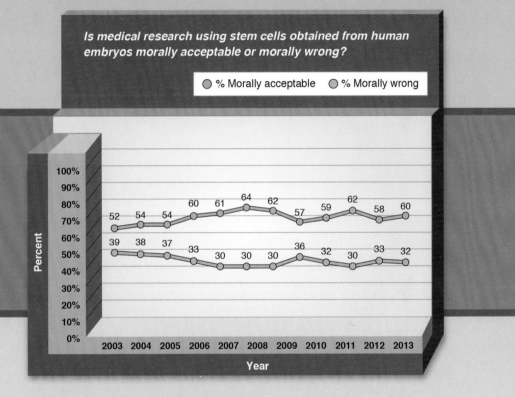

Is medical research using stem cells obtained from human embryos morally acceptable or morally wrong?

○ % Morally acceptable   ○ % Morally wrong

Source: Gallup, "Stem Cell Research," 2013. www.gallup.com.

Not Yet a Person

Embryonic stem cell research does involve the destruction of human embryos; however, this is not the same as destroying a person. Thus, it is ethically permissible. The early embryo that is used for research is a collection of cells with the potential to become a person; however, it is not yet a person. The Ethics Committee of the American Society for Reproductive Medicine explains this distinction. It points out that the early embryo has no nervous system and still has a good chance of becoming nonviable or of splitting into twins. Thus, it cannot be argued that this early embryo is an individual person. Instead, says the committee, "the embryo has a status distinctly different from adults and children." It argues that the embryo is "a potential human being worthy of respect but not entitled to the same rights as persons."[36] The committee—like many other groups in favor of stem cell research—believes that it is ethical to use the embryo for research, as long as it is shown respect. This means obtaining consent to use it and using it in ways that may benefit society.

> "Embryonic stem cells have a virtually unlimited future. . . . It would be truly immoral if the nation *does not* move to capitalize on the tantalizing potential of these new medical treatments."[35]
>
> —Daniel Perry, executive director of the Alliance for Aging Research.

Embryos from Fertility Clinics

Embryonic stem cell research depends on a steady supply of embryos, and one ethical way to obtain these is to use excess embryos created in fertility clinics. When patients undergo in vitro fertilization at a clinic, excess embryos are usually produced. Surveys show that many people are uncomfortable with destroying the excess embryos or with allowing other in vitro patients to adopt them. Because of this, many are simply left in storage—for years. Seattle University law professor Julie Shapiro says, "There are at least tens of thousands if not hundreds of thousands of frozen embryos in little freezers all over the world, and no one knows quite what to do with them."[37]

Clinics cannot store all these embryos indefinitely. So why not use them to benefit society? The idea of leaving them in storage in perpetuity is far more unethical than giving them a purpose that will help so many people. As researcher John Harris says, "Faced with the opportunity to use resources for a beneficial purpose when the alternative is that those resources are wasted, we have powerful moral reasons to avoid waste and do good instead."[38] In the case of embryos left over from fertility treatments, destroying them would be a waste—with no benefit to anyone. In contrast, donating excess embryos for research offers the potential for good, because embryonic stem cell research is likely to benefit society.

Research reveals that many people who have excess embryos left over from fertility treatment are in favor of donating them for stem cell research. According to a study by the Stanford University School of Medicine about donation of excess embryos for research, "Many couples were very relieved to have the option to donate their embryos for research and to participate in the field of stem cell research."[39] For example, in an online comment to an article about embryo donation, Carla says that she donated her excess embryos because of the benefit to research. She says, "After our daughter was born we decided that we had been blessed with our two children and that we should donate our remaining 5 embryos to research. We felt strongly that we should give something back to the program and we have not regretted this decision."[40]

Public Funding for Stem Cell Research

Not only should donation and research be encouraged, but the government should provide funding for embryonic stem cell research. Because embryonic stem cell research has the potential to alleviate so much suffering, the government has an ethical duty to use its great power to help realize that potential. Private funding is important, but government funding is the most effective way to stimulate research. It will help researchers achieve the breakthroughs that will allow them to successfully use stem cells to cure diseases and create replacement tissues and organs. Journalist Tyler Cabot points out that the power of government support has enabled the United States to achieve other important goals. For example, he says, "It took a good deal of work, but the country demanded we figure out a way to treat AIDS, and what was once a death sentence is now a chronic condition. [President Barack] Obama put billions of dollars toward clean energy, and now we are on the cusp of a burgeoning electric car and battery industry."[41] In the same way, he believes that tremendous progress could be made if the government invests money and support in embryonic stem cell research.

Although embryonic stem cell research involves the destruction of an early embryo, the research has the potential to greatly benefit society, and this benefit is more important than the destruction of the embryo. Embryonic stem cell research is ethical and should be encouraged by government funding and facilitated by the donation of excess embryos from fertility clinics.

Embryonic Stem Cell Research Is Not Ethical

"Taking the life of a human being at any stage in development for research is ethically wrong. The embryos that are being destroyed are more than just tissue. These unborn children already are alive."

—Right to Life of Michigan, an organization that works to protect life at all stages, believes that embryonic stem cell research is wrong.

Right to Life of Michigan, "Sacrificed Without Consent: Taking from the Unborn, Ending Lives," 2013. www.rtl.org.

Consider these questions as you read:

1. Do you agree that it is unethical to destroy even an early embryo? Why or why not?
2. How strong is the argument that researchers can conduct effective research without using embryonic stem cells? Explain your opinion.
3. Which pieces of evidence in this discussion provide the strongest support for the argument that embryonic stem cell research is not ethical? Why do you think they are the strongest?

Editor's note: The discussion that follows presents common arguments made in support of this perspective, reinforced by facts, quotes, and examples taken from various sources.

Every human being starts out as an embryo. The embryo is created when a sperm fertilizes an egg, thus combining the genetic material of two people and creating an entirely new cell. The fertilized egg begins to grow rapidly, and within a few days it has about 150 cells. This early embryo—called a blastocyst—is what researchers destroy in order to obtain embryonic stem cells for research. However, even though it is not yet fully developed, the embryo is the beginning of a human being, with its own unique combination of genetic material. Using it for research means the destruction of a beginning human life and thus is unethical.

The Embryo Deserves Respect

From the moment it is created, an embryo is a potential human being, and it should be given the same respect as any other human being. Destroying it for research is wrong, no matter how small it is or what the potential benefits of the research are. Peter Saunders, a doctor and the CEO of the Christian Medical Fellowship, argues that every embryo is a potential human being. He says, "Any biology textbook tells us that human development is a continuous process beginning with fertilization." Even when it is tiny, he says, "biologically the human embryo is undoubtedly human; it has human chromosomes derived from human gametes [reproductive cells]. It is also alive, exhibiting movement, respiration, sensitivity, growth, reproduction, excretion and nutrition."[42]

> "Biologically the human embryo is undoubtedly human."[42]
>
> —Peter Saunders, a doctor and the CEO of the Christian Medical Fellowship.

While the embryo does not have all the characteristics of a human, it will become a human and should be given the same respect. Advocates of embryonic stem cell research argue that this research has the potential to benefit society; however, these possible benefits simply do not justify the destruction of the embryo for research. Destroying an embryo is morally and ethically wrong, no matter the reason.

Other Methods Can Be Used

In fact, there is no evidence that embryonic stem cell research has yielded any medical benefits. Scientists have failed to successfully treat any disease using embryonic stem cells or to use embryonic stem cells to create any replacement organs that can be used in humans. Says David Prentice, cell biologist and senior fellow for life sciences at the Family Research Council:

In the 27 years since the advent of embryonic stem-cell research in 1981, scientists have still not demonstrated the ability to control the cells and their attendant risk of tumor formation, inappropriate tissue growth and immune rejection, and the leading researchers continue to note that it will be decades at best before embryonic stem cells might possibly be used for patients.[43]

Why continue to destroy human embryos for stem cells when medical science already has a proven alternative in adult stem cells? These cells are found in many tissues and organs, including the brain and skin, and they have the ability to grow into different cell types depending on what part of the body they are in. Prentice says, "Hundreds of published references document the ability of adult stem cells from bone marrow, umbilical cord blood and even fat tissue in effectively alleviating symptoms of dozens of diseases."[44] Clearly, the ethical choice is to focus on improving these adult stem cell treatments and making them more widely available.

In 2012 researchers reported on one successful treatment created with adult stem cells. They conducted a study on twenty-five patients who had been left with damaged heart muscle after heart attacks. Eight of the patients were given conventional treatments such as medication and exercise recommendations, and after twelve months most of these patients had no reduction in damage. The other seventeen patients received stem cells that came from small pieces of their own heart tissue. The researchers report that in these patients, there was an almost 50 percent reduction in damage after twelve months. This reduction is significant and has been highly beneficial for these patients. For example, one study participant, Fred Lesikar of California, says that the scars from his heart attack had reduced his heart function by more than 30 percent. He says, "The doctors treating me told me that there was no way to repair a heart damaged by a heart attack." However, as a result of the stem cell treatment, he says, "Today I'm feeling super—better than I did before the heart attack."[45]

Embryos from Fertility Clinics

Some of the embryos used in stem cell research are excess embryos discarded from fertility clinics. The fact that these embryos are no longer

Embryonic stem cell research is an extremely controversial issue in the United States. Many people strongly believe that it is unethical and that it should not be supported by the government. As a result of such opposition, government funding for this type of research has been limited. This chart shows funding by the National Institutes of Health for both embryonic and non-embryonic stem cell research from 2002 through 2012. It reveals that most federal funds go to non-embryonic research.

Year	Embryonic (Dollars in millions)	Non–embryonic (Dollars in millions)
2002	$10.1	$170.9
2003	$20.3	$190.7
2004	$24.3	$203.2
2005	$39.6	$199.4
2006	$37.8	$206.1
2007	$42.1	$203.5
2008	$88.1	$297.2
2009	$119.9	$339.3
2010	$125.5	$340.8
2011	$123.0	$394.6
2012	$146.5	$504.0

Source: National Institutes of Health, "NIH Stem Cell Research Funding, FY 2002–2012," 2013. http://stemcells.nih.gov.

needed by the patients at these clinics does not justify their destruction for research. Micheline Mathews-Roth, associate professor of medicine at Harvard Medical School, says, "The suggestion that we use leftover embryos from fertility clinics because 'they are going to be destroyed anyway' is discrimination against a class of human beings—the very young." She points out that the embryos do not even have to be destroyed, because many couples who are unable to create their own embryos would gratefully adopt them. She says, "We should offer these extra embryos to infertile couples to implant and allow them to be born, and not kill them either by experimentation or by disposal."[46] According to the CDC's most recent statistics, 6.7 million women in the United States between the ages of fifteen and forty-four are unable to get pregnant or carry a baby to term. Embryo adoption would give some of these women the chance to have a child when it is otherwise impossible.

One mother and blogger talks about how she is opposed to research using excess embryos. She insists:

> "The search for treatments and cures need not include the destruction of innocent, vulnerable human embryos."[49]
>
> —The Right to Life of Michigan, an organization opposed to the destruction of human embryos, including for stem cell research.

> I do believe that life begins at conception . . . and the embryos growing in a petri dish, or frozen in a vat, have an excellent chance of growing in to a *unique* and sacred human being in 9-months time. . . . I would . . . have a difficult time donating any of my embryos for research. Even though my very own father is suffering from Parkinson's Disease, and I know *very well* that 'the cure' may lie in stem cell research, it would haunt me forever that I may have robbed my child (or children) of a chance at life.[47]

No Public Funding

Because embryonic stem cell research is unethical, the government should not encourage it by providing funding for it. The NIH and other federal agencies give various types of researchers millions of dollars in funding every year in order to help support and advance their research. However, giving researchers funds to use for embryonic stem cell research sends society the message that embryo destruction is acceptable. In addition, it encourages an increasing number of researchers to participate in this research, resulting in increased embryo destruction. Overall, as the Right to Life of Michigan explains, "by providing federal funds for research on embryonic stem cells, the NIH is promoting the destruction of innocent lives."[48]

While some researchers argue that embryonic stem cell research is necessary because it has the potential to benefit society, the fact is that there are equally effective research alternatives. The Right to Life of Michigan insists, "The search for treatments and cures need not include the destruction of innocent, vulnerable human embryos. Stem cell research can move forward, alternatives to human embryonic stem cells exist."[49] Embryonic stem cell research is not necessary or ethical and should be not be conducted or receive funding from the federal government.

Chapter Four

Should the United States Change Its Organ Donation Policies?

The United States Needs to Change Its Organ Donation Policies

- Younger patients should have higher priority than older patients for receiving organs.
- Personal behavior should be considered in determining who has priority for organs.
- Allowing payments for donated organs would increase supply and reduce the black market trade.
- Instituting presumed consent is an ethical way to solve the problem of organ shortages.

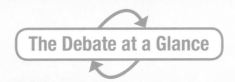

The Debate at a Glance

The United States Should Not Change Its Organ Donation Policies

- The US organ donation system is effective and ethical.
- Everybody on the organ waiting list should have an equal chance of receiving an organ.
- Financial compensation for organ donation is unethical.
- Presumed consent is unethical and unnecessary.

The United States Needs to Change Its Organ Donation Policies

"With so many lives at stake, we cannot afford to simply continue our current insufficient approach to organ procurement. It is time to try something new."

—Carl Cohen, a professor of philosophy at the University of Michigan.

Carl Cohen, quoted in Stephen Holland, ed., *Arguing About Bioethics*. New York: Routledge, 2012, p. 274.

Consider these questions as you read:

1. Do you agree that younger people will get greater benefit than older people from donated organs? Why or why not?
2. Can you think of any possible harm that might result from allowing people to be paid for donating organs? Explain.
3. How strong is the argument that allowing financial compensation for organs would reduce the black market? Explain.

Editor's note: The discussion that follows presents common arguments made in support of this perspective, reinforced by facts, quotes, and examples taken from various sources.

Eleven-year-old Sarah Murnaghan was born with cystic fibrosis, and the disease eventually destroyed her lungs—meaning that without a new pair, she would die. Murnaghan was placed on the US organ donation waiting list for children's lungs. However, children's lungs rarely become available, and after about eighteen months on the list, she still had not received lungs. Her condition continued to deteriorate. In an attempt to save their daughter's life, Murnaghan's parents filed a federal lawsuit in June 2013 arguing that the organ donation policy discriminates against children by not allowing them to receive adult lungs. They argued that their daughter should be eligible to receive

52

a pair of adult lungs, which become available much more frequently and can be used for children. Their challenge was successful, and that same month Murnaghan underwent two transplants of adult lungs, the second of which was successful.

Ideally, everybody who needs an organ would get one, but in the United States there are not enough available organs. So a system has been developed to decide who gets priority. Murnaghan's case highlights the dire need to rethink this system, which does not provide the most ethical solution for procuring organs or allocating them for donation.

Changing Who Gets Priority

At present, the main factors influencing organ allocation are blood type and body size, the severity of the patient's condition, how long the patient has been waiting, and the distance between the donor's hospital and the patient's hospital (since organs must be transplanted within hours of removal). This is not the most ethical system, because it ignores other important factors such as how much benefit the patient is likely to get from the organ and whether or not the patient is responsible for his or her own organ failure.

One important change that should be made is to give priority to younger people in order to maximize the benefit of scarce organs. The main reason that younger people can make better use of donations is that they are likely to live longer than older people after a transplant. For example, a twenty-year-old has far more potential years of life left than a seventy-year-old. In addition, a younger body is more likely to successfully accept the transplanted organ. Explains *New York Times* writer Paula Span, "Younger recipients have greater physiologic reserve to aid in the arduous recovery; older ones face higher risk of subsequent kidney failure, stroke, diabetes and other diseases."[50]

Current policies also make no distinction between people who need organs because of their own bad choices and those who did nothing to cause their own organ failure. For example, some people experience liver failure because of an illness out of their control; however, others destroy their livers by repeatedly choosing to drink large quantities of alcohol. It is unethical to allow a person who is responsible for his or her own organ failure the same chance of a new organ as everybody else. Instead, patients who have not chosen harmful behavior should have a higher priority for organs.

Payment for Donated Organs

In addition to changing organ allocation policies, the United States also needs to increase supply by changing the way organs are donated. The most obvious way to increase the availability of organs is to pay healthy people to donate them. A living person can donate a kidney, bone marrow, and part of the liver. Given the dire need for organs, it would be unethical not to increase supply by offering financial compensation.

> "The organ shortage can be solved by paying living donors."[51]
>
> —Alex Tabarrok, a professor of economics at George Mason University and director of research for the Independent Institute.

At present, Iran is the only country where financial compensation for organs is legal, and this policy has successfully increased organ supply. Under government regulation there, kidney donors receive an estimated $2,000 to $4,000, some of which comes from the government and some from the kidney recipient or a charitable organization. Alex Tabarrok, professor of economics at George Mason University and director of research for the Independent Institute, maintains that this system has been extremely successful. He says, "Only one country, Iran, has eliminated the shortage of transplant organs—and only Iran has a working and legal payment system for organ donation." He concludes that Iran's system demonstrates that "the organ shortage can be solved by paying living donors. The Iranian system began in 1988 and eliminated the shortage of kidneys by 1999."[51]

Financial compensation for organs would have the added benefit of reducing the thriving black market for organs, which preys on poor,

Current Donation Policies Do Not Meet Demand

Leaving current organ donation policies in place would be unethical. The US organ donation system cannot keep pace with the desperate and rising need for organs. As this graph shows, the number of people donating and the number of transplants being performed is increasing at a much slower rate than the number of people awaiting organ transplants.

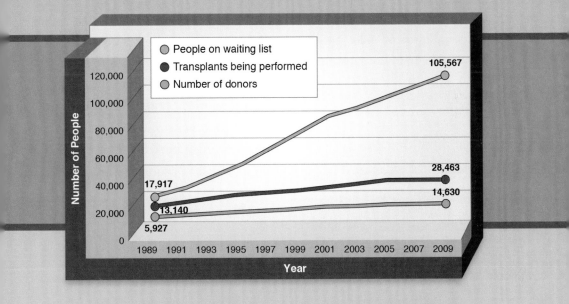

Source: US Department of Health and Human Services, "About Donation and Transplantation: The Need Is Real; Data," no date. http://organdonor.gov.

desperate people. Psychiatrist and author Sally Satel explains that even though it is illegal in almost every part of the world to sell organs, there is such a high demand for them that a black market has been created. She says that in this market, poor and vulnerable people donate their organs without receiving adequate compensation or medical care. In her opinion, this abuse will continue as long as there is a shortage of organs, because dying people who need organs will pay for them on the black market. She says, "Many people without a donor . . . will follow that survival instinct to foreign lands, despite the sickening knowledge that their new organ might come from an executed prisoner in China or an illiterate laborer in India."[52] By paying people legally instead, the black market could be reduced because demand would be met legally. It is unethical not to institute this proven solution.

Institute Presumed Consent

Another way to solve the current organ shortage in the United States is to rewrite the law to enact a system of presumed consent. With the current system, donors or their family must expressly consent to donation. This means that many organs are wasted simply because many people never make their wishes clear before they die. Under a presumed consent law, people would be presumed to have consented to donation unless they opt out, or expressly state that they do not want to be donors.

> "Numerous polls and surveys show that most Americans are willing to be organ donors upon their deaths."[53]
>
> —Arthur Caplan, a bioethicist.

Bioethicist Arthur Caplan argues in favor of presumed consent for organ donations, citing consistent public support for such a system. He says, "Numerous polls and surveys show that most Americans are willing to be organ donors upon their deaths. Yet the system we have in place now— using donor cards and driver's license check-offs—to permit people to let their wishes be known does not capture the altruism and goodwill that is out there." There are many ways that goodwill does not get translated into donation. For example, he says, "cards and licenses get lost or misplaced or those who sign them fail to talk about their wishes with their families meaning that organs are buried or cremated when they could be saving lives."[53] There is evidence from other countries that presumed consent is an effective way to increase donation. For example, Spain instituted presumed consent in 1979 and has the highest rate of donation in the world.

According to the US Department of Health and Human Services, the gap between donors and people who need organs continues to widen. It says, "Right now, there are more than enough people waiting for an organ to fill a large football stadium twice over."[54] It is unethical to allow so many people to suffer when there are alternatives. The United States needs to change its organ donation policies in order to address this problem.

The United States Should Not Change Its Organ Donation Policies

"[In the United States] both state and federal legislation has been put in place to provide the safest and most equitable system for allocation, distribution, and transplantation of donated organs."

—US Department of Health and Human Services, the government agency that works to protect the health of all Americans.

US Department of Health and Human Services, "Legislation and Policy," Organdonor.gov. www.organdonor.gov.

Consider these questions as you read:

1. Can you think of an example when an organ donation might be more beneficial to an elderly person than a younger one? Explain.
2. How strong is the argument that financial compensation for organ donation is unethical? Explain.
3. How persuasive is the argument that the United States should not change its organ donation policies? Which arguments provide the strongest support for this perspective?

Editor's note: The discussion that follows presents common arguments made in support of this perspective, reinforced by facts, quotes, and examples taken from various sources.

The US government faces a difficult job in regulating the donation and allocation of organs in a population of more than 300 million people. On any given day thousands of people await word of a compatible organ that can make life more bearable or in many cases mean the difference between life and death. This national list of people who need organs includes patients all over the country, in varying states of health, and in need of numerous different organs, including kidneys, hearts, and lungs.

The unfortunate reality is that while most people who face this issue believe that they or their loved one are the most deserving of an organ, there are simply not enough organs for everybody who needs them.

To deal with this problem, a great deal of thought has gone into evaluating different policies and creating the most ethical system of allocation possible. The United Network for Organ Sharing—the organization responsible for coordinating transplant policies—explains, "Organ allocation policies are designed as equitable as possible while making the best use of the limited number of donor organs."[55] This system works. Every day an average of seventy-nine people are successfully matched up with donations and receive organ transplants.

Equal Opportunity

One way the system stays fair is by treating everybody equally. Some critics believe that since organs are scarce in the United States, transplant priority should be given to those who are likely to receive the greatest benefit, such as young people who have more potential years of life left. Others argue that people who have caused their own organ failure through irresponsible lifestyle choices should have lower priority. However, this would be unfair. The only ethical way for the transplant system to stay fair is to treat everybody equally, regardless of their age or their personal circumstances. Marie Budev is medical director of the lung transplant program at the Cleveland Clinic. She says, "We feel that everyone should have a chance."[56]

The US transplant system accomplishes the goal of equal treatment by using the same rules for matching organs in every case it oversees. People needing donations all have to wait on a list. Organ allocation is done by using an established set of criteria that includes factors such as blood type and the distance between the donor's hospital and the patient's hospital. Value judgments such as who might get the greatest benefit from the organ are not part of the process because they would make it unfair. For example, it would be unethical to assume that an elderly person's life is worth less than that of somebody younger. Although an older person might not live for as many more years as a younger transplant recipient, they value their remaining years just as much as a young person. "Many of these older patients can transition to an even older age while maintaining a very good quality of life. Why would we deny someone that opportunity?"[57] says Mandeep Mehra, executive director of the Center for Advanced Heart Disease at Brigham and Women's Hospital in Boston. In fact, some people argue that an elderly patient who receives a transplant might get more out of their remaining years than a younger person. In a study of five hundred heart transplant patients of various ages published in the *Journal of Heart and Lung Transplantation* in May 2012, researchers state that patients aged sixty and older reported greater satisfaction with their quality of life and less depression and stress than younger patients.

Paying for Organs Is Wrong

Clearly, the problems with the organ transplant system are rooted in the fact that there are too many people needing too few organs. This has led to calls for a system of financial compensation for donation, in hopes of increasing supply. However, such a policy would be unethical because it would result in harm to vulnerable people in need of money. At present, most organ donors make donations for altruistic reasons. Renal physician Jeremy Chapman argues that donation must remain that way. He uses the example of kidney donation and warns, "The moment that money is introduced to buy a kidney from a vendor, the nature of the exchange and the motivation changes, and with that change come dangerous consequences for both parties."[58] The major consequence is that donors are no longer those who want to help others by donating but rather those people who need the money. Allowing people to sell their organs means that the poor and vulnerable can be coerced into selling without fully

> "The moment that money is introduced to buy a kidney from a vendor, the nature of the exchange and the motivation changes, and with that change come dangerous consequences for both parties."[58]
>
> —Jeremy Chapman, a renal physician.

The US Organ Donation System Works Better than Most

While some people criticize the US organ donation system as ineffective, an examination of worldwide data reveals that the United States actually has a high rate of organ donation and transplantation compared with other countries. In the United States in 2012 more than seventy-five organs were transplanted per million people. Most other countries had lower rates of transplantation.

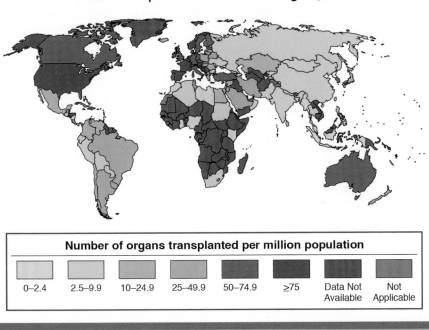

Global Transplantation Activities of Organs, 2012

Number of organs transplanted per million population

| 0–2.4 | 2.5–9.9 | 10–24.9 | 25–49.9 | 50–74.9 | ≥75 | Data Not Available | Not Applicable |

Source: Global Observatory on Donation and Transplantation, "Global Transplantation Activities of Solid Organs, 2012." www.transplant-observatory.org.

understanding the health risks and without receiving adequate care and compensation.

Medical anthropologist Monir Moniruzzaman has spent time in Bangladesh learning the stories of poor people there who are so desperate for money that they have resorted to selling a kidney. His investigation reveals that in most cases these people were taken advantage of by brokers who did not warn them about the health risks such as bleeding and infection, did not offer adequate medical treatment, and did not even provide adequate compensation. "Most of them didn't even know what an organ is, or its function,"[59] Moniruzzaman said.

Presumed Consent Is Unethical

Another proposed change to the US organ donation system is to institute presumed consent, whereby all citizens are presumed to be donors unless they state otherwise. However, such a policy would also be unethical because it would mean that doctors might take organs against a person's wishes—for example, if a person is opposed to donation but fails to make his or her wishes known or if the document with his or her wishes becomes lost. Instead, Dorry L. Segev, associate professor of surgery at the Johns Hopkins University School of Medicine, says a better solution is to educate people so that they will willingly give consent for donation. He says, "We need to foster more awareness of transplantation and transplant issues to procure more organs for lifesaving transplants rather than force people to donate their relatives' organs if they fail to opt-out before death."[60]

> "We need to foster more awareness of transplantation and transplant issues to procure more organs for lifesaving transplants rather than force people to donate their relatives' organs if they fail to opt-out before death."[60]
>
> —Dorry L. Segev, an associate professor of surgery at the Johns Hopkins University School of Medicine.

Education and awareness, not presumed consent, is one of the reasons that some other countries such as Spain have high organ donation rates. Although Spain does have a policy of presumed consent, in practice doctors there speak with family members and obtain consent before taking organs for transplant. Kieran Healy, author of *Last Best Gifts: Altruism and the Market for Human Blood and Organs*, explains, "Spain's success is due to effective management of the transplant system."[61] Segev reports that in Spain there are dedicated transplant specialists at every hospital who screen for potential donors and approach families to talk about donation. He believes this focus on education and awareness is the reason Spain has a high rate of donation.

The United States has developed an organ donation system that is both ethical and effective. According to a 2013 report by ABC News, the United States is actually one of the most successful countries in the world when it comes to organ donation. It has the fourth highest donation rate and leads the world in transplant rates. US organ donation policies do not need to be changed.

Source Notes

Overview: Biomedical Ethics

1. Quoted in Torsten Ove, "The Next Page/Before Tuskegee, the Guatemala Experiment: A Pitt Legend's Research Is Under Scrutiny," *Pittsburgh Post-Gazette*, June 12, 2011. www.post-gazette.com.
2. Quoted in White House, "President Obama Establishes New Presidential Commission for the Study of Bioethical Issues, Names Commission Leadership," November 24, 2009. www.whitehouse.gov.

Chapter One: Should Physician-Assisted Suicide Be Legal?

3. Quoted in Melissa Barber, "Dr. Donald Low: Legalize Death with Dignity," Death with Dignity National Center, October 2, 2013. www.deathwithdignity.org.
4. Quoted in CBC News, "SARS Doctor Donald Low's Posthumous Plea," September 24, 2013. www.cbcnews.ca.
5. Nora Miller, "Experiences of a Dying Patient," Death with Dignity National Center, October 14, 2011. www.deathwithdignity.org.
6. Quoted in Reed Karaim, "Assisted Suicide," *CQ Researcher*, May 17, 2013. www.cqresearcher.com.
7. Timothy E. Quill, "Physicians Should 'Assist in Suicide' When It Is Appropriate," *Journal of Law, Medicine & Ethics*, Spring 2012, p. 58.
8. Netherlands Ministry of Foreign Affairs, "FAQ: Euthanasia 2010," 2010. www.patientsrightscouncil.org.
9. American Medical Association, "Opinion 2.211—Physician-Assisted Suicide," June 1996. www.ama-assn.org.
10. Quoted in Jamie Komarnicki, "Doctors Debate Physician-Assisted Suicide: Canadian Medical Association Meeting," *Calgary Herald* (Alberta, Canada), August 20, 2013. www.calgaryherald.com.
11. David Blazer, "Sunday Dialogue: Choosing How We Die," *New York Times*, March 27, 2013. www.nytimes.com.

12. American Medical Association, "Opinion 2.211—Physician-Assisted Suicide."

13. Center to Advance Palliative Care and the National Palliative Care Research Center, "America's Care of Serious Illness: A State-by-State Report Card on Access to Palliative Care in Our Nation's Hospitals," 2011. http://reportcard.capc.org.

14. Mary E. Harned, "The Dangers of Assisted Suicide: No Longer Theoretical," *Defending Life 2012*, Americans United for Life, 2012. www.aul.org.

15. Kenneth Stevens, "Assisted Suicide," *Hamilton (MT) Ravalli Republic*, November 24, 2012. www.ravallirepublic.com.

16. Patrick Lee, "Say No to Physician Assisted Suicide," *Cato Unbound*, December 2012. www.cato-unbound.org.

17. José Pereira, "Legalizing Euthanasia or Assisted Suicide: The Illusion of Safeguards and Controls," *Current Oncology*, vol. 18, no. 2, 2011. www.current-oncology.com.

Chapter Two: Should Society Allow Genetic Testing?

18. Lee Gutkind and Pagan Kennedy, *An Immense New Power to Heal: The Promise of Personalized Medicine*. Pittsburgh, PA: In Fact, 2012, p. 38.

19. Quoted in Ginny Allain, "Personalized Medicine," *Medical Laboratory Observer*, July 2012. www.mlo-online.com.

20. Gutkind and Kennedy, *An Immense New Power to Heal*.

21. Angelina Jolie, "My Medical Choice," *New York Times*, May 14, 2013. www.nytimes.com.

22. Jill Uchiyama, comment on *Slate*, "What Did You Learn from 23and Me?," April 23, 2013. www.slate.com.

23. Katherine Wasson et al., "Primary Care Patients' Views and Decisions About, Experience of and Reactions to Direct-to-Consumer Genetic Testing: A Longitudinal Study," *Journal of Community Genetics*, October 2013. www.springer.com.

24. Quoted in Wasson et al., "Primary Care Patients' Views and Decisions About, Experience of and Reactions to Direct-to-Consumer Genetic Testing."

25. Megan Pline, comment on EverydayFamily, "Did You Opt for Pre-natal Genetic Testing? Why or Why Not? I'm Torn on the Idea!," September 28, 2013. www.facebook.com.

26. Jennifer Kentfield, comment on EverydayFamily, "Did You Opt for Prenatal Genetic Testing?"

27. Quoted in Jasmeet Sidhu, "How to Buy a Daughter," *Slate*, September 14, 2012. www.slate.com.

28. Quoted in Sidhu, "How to Buy a Daughter."

29. Daniel Allott and Neumary George, "Eugenic Abortion 2.0: A New Blood Test Could Zero Out the Disabled Unborn in the 21st Century," *American Spectator*, May 2013. http://spectator.org.

30. Carolyn Y. Johnson, "As Down Detection Gets Easier, Choices Harder," *Boston Globe*, March 24, 2013. www.bostonglobe.com.

31. Bruce Grierson, 'To Know or Not to Know," *Psychology Today*, May/June 2011. www.psychologytoday.com.

32. National Institutes of Health, "What Is Direct-to-Consumer Genetic Testing?," *Genetics Home Reference*, November 12, 2013. http://ghr.nlm.nih.gov.

33. National Institutes of Health, "What Is Direct-to-Consumer Genetic Testing?"

Chapter Three: Is Embryonic Stem Cell Research Ethical?

34. Americans for Cures Foundation, "Stem Cell Facts." www.americansforcures.org.

35. Quoted in Micheline Mathews-Roth, "Stem Cell Research: An NPR Special Report," National Public Radio, November 22, 2013. www.npr.org.

36. Ethics Committee of the American Society for Reproductive Medicine, "Donating Embryos for Human Embryonic Stem Cell (hESC) Research: A Committee Opinion," *Fertility and Sterility*, October 2013.

37. Quoted in Bonnie Rochman, "Gingrich Wants Scrutiny of IVF Clinics: Why That's Not the Worst Idea," *Time*, January 13, 2012. http://healthland.time.com.

38. Quoted in Stephen Holland, ed., *Arguing About Bioethics*. New York: Routledge, 2012, p. 50.

39. Quoted in Krista Conger, "New Approach to IVF Embryo Donation Lets People Weigh Decision," Stanford School of Medicine, April 7, 2011. http://med.stanford.edu.

40. Carla, comment on Claire Thompson, "What to Do with Excess Embryos," *Daily Life*, March 32, 2013. www.dailylife.com.au.

41. Tyler Cabot, "Whatever Happened to Stem Cells?," *Esquire*, April 2013, p. 120.

42. Peter Saunders, "The Moral Status of the Human Embryo: When Is a Person a Person?," LifeNews.com, July 3, 2013. www.lifenews.com.

43. David Prentice, comment on *The Survival Doctor* (blog), "Embryonic Stem-Cell Research: Experts Debate Pros and Cons," February 14, 2013. www.thesurvivaldoctor.com.

44. Prentice, comment on *The Survival Doctor* (blog), "Embryonic Stem-Cell Research."

45. Quoted in Ryan Jaslow, "Stem Cells Heal Heart Attack Scars, Regrow Healthy Muscle," CBS News, February 14, 2012. www.cbsnews.com.

46. Mathews-Roth, "Stem Cell Research."

47. *The Amazing Trips* (blog), "Playing God," October 5, 2007. http://theamazingtrips.blogspot.com.

48. Right to Life of Michigan, "Sacrificed Without Consent: Taking from the Unborn, Ending Lives," 2013. www.rtl.org.

49. Right to Life of Michigan, "Sacrificed Without Consent."

Chapter Four: Should the United States Change Its Organ Donation Policies?

50. Paula Span, "Who Should Receive Organ Transplants?," *New York Times*, January 8, 2013. www.nytimes.com.

51. Alex Tabarrok, "The Meat Market," *Wall Street Journal*, January 8, 2010. www.wsj.com.

52. Sally Satel, "Is It Ever Right to Buy or Sell Human Organs? Yes," *New Internationalist*, October 2010. www.newint.org.

53. Arthur Caplan, comment on *New York Times*, "Should Laws Push for Organ Donation?," May 2, 2010. www.nytimes.com.

54. US Department of Health and Human Services, "About Donation and Transplantation: The Need Is Real; Data." http://organdonor.gov.

55. United Network for Organ Sharing, "Policies." www.transplantliving.org.

56. Quoted in Span, "Who Should Receive Organ Transplants?"

57. Quoted in Judith Graham, "Heart Transplants for Older Patients," *New York Times*, April 30, 2012. www.nytimes.com.

58. Jeremy Chapman, "Is It Ever Right to Buy or Sell Human Organs? No," *New Internationalist*, October 2010. www.newint.org.

59. Quoted in Lee Dye, "Organs for Sale: Impoverished Bangladeshis Try to Sell Kidneys on Black Market, End Up Poor and Ill," ABC News, March 16, 2012. http://abcnews.go.com.

60. Quoted in Johns Hopkins Medicine, "Presumed Consent Not Answer to Solving Organ Shortage in U.S., Researchers Say," November 29, 2011. www.hopkinsmedicine.org.

61. Kieran Healy, comment on *New York Times*, "Should Laws Push for Organ Donation?"

Biomedical Ethics Facts

Physician-Assisted Suicide

- According to a 2011 Gallup poll of 1,018 Americans, 45 percent believe physician-assisted suicide is morally acceptable, and 48 percent believe it is morally wrong.
- According to the Oregon Public Health Division, in 2012, 115 lethal prescriptions were written under Oregon's Death with Dignity Act, and they were written by sixty-one physicians.
- According to the Washington State Department of Health, of those people who used the state's Death with Dignity Act in 2012, 94 percent were concerned with losing autonomy, 90 percent that they would be less able to participate in activities that make life enjoyable, and 84 percent about a loss of dignity.
- According to a 2010 poll of 2,340 adult Americans by Harris Interactive, 70 percent believe that people who are terminally ill and in great pain should have the right to choose to end their lives.
- Deaths under Oregon's Death with Dignity Act have increased from sixteen in 1998 to seventy-seven in 2012.

Genetic Testing

- According to a survey conducted by Johns Hopkins University and reported in *Genetic Testing and Molecular Biomarkers* in 2013, of 1,046 people who chose to undergo genetic testing, 91 percent did it to learn about potential future diseases.
- According to *USA Today* in 2012, between 60 and 90 percent of women who receive a prenatal Down syndrome diagnosis choose to end their pregnancy.
- Every time two carriers of cystic fibrosis conceive, there is a 25 percent chance of passing the disease to their children and a 50 percent chance that the child will be a carrier of the cystic fibrosis gene.

- In a study reported in the *Journal of Genetic Counseling* in February 2012, of 382 family and internal medicine doctors, 38.7 percent were aware of direct-to-consumer genetic testing, and 15 percent felt prepared to answer questions from their patients about these tests.
- In *Familial Cancer* in September 2013, researchers reported that in a study of 370 people with hereditary breast and ovarian cancer, 43 percent would consider using preimplantation genetic diagnosis to avoid passing the disease on to their children.
- A study by Robert Green, a researcher in the Genetics Department at Harvard Medical School, finds that people who discover they have the gene associated with Alzheimer's are five times more likely than the average person to buy long-term-care insurance.

Embryonic Stem Cell Research

- In a 2010 Harris Interactive poll of 2,113 adults, 75 percent said they believe that stem cell research should be allowed as long as the parents of the embryo give their permission and the embryo would otherwise be destroyed.
- Between 2001 and 2009 federal funding for embryonic stem cell research was only allowed for research involving twenty-one government-approved stem cell lines.
- In a 2013 survey of 4,006 adults, the Pew Research Center found that only 22 percent of respondents believe that embryonic stem cell research is morally wrong.
- According to the NIH, in 2012 the agency provided $146.5 million in funding for human embryonic stem cell research and $504 million for nonembryonic stem cell research.

Organ Transplantation

- According to the Global Observatory on Donation and Transplantation, in 2011 approximately 112,600 organs were transplanted worldwide, an increase of 5.4 percent over 2010.

- The US Department of Health and Human Services reports that more than 100 million people in the United States are signed up to be organ donors.
- According to the US Department of Health and Human Services, each day in the United States an average of 79 people receive organ transplants. In 2012, a total of 28,051 people received organ transplants.
- In a 2012 NPR–Thomson Reuters health poll of three thousand American adults, 41 percent said they felt that cash compensation for organ donation would be acceptable.
- According to a 2012 National Public Radio report, since it became possible to perform a living kidney donation in the 1950s, more than one hundred thousand people have donated a kidney.

Related Organizations and Websites

American Medical Association (AMA)
515 N. State St.
Chicago, IL 60610
phone: (800) 621-8335
website: www.ama-assn.org

The AMA is a national association representing American physicians. It works to improve public health. The association has information and position statements about various biomedical ethics topics on its website.

American Society of Law, Medicine & Ethics (ASLME)
765 Commonwealth Ave., Suite 1634
Boston, MA 02215
phone: (617) 262-4990 • fax: (617) 437-7596
e-mail: info@aslme.org • website: www.aslme.org

The ASLME is a nonprofit educational organization that provides information about law, medicine, and ethics. It works to protect public health, reduce health disparities, and improve care. Its website contains information about numerous biomedical issues, including genetic testing and physician-assisted suicide. It also publishes the *Journal of Law, Medicine & Ethics* and the *American Journal of Law & Medicine*.

Dignity in Dying
181 Oxford St.
London W1D 2JT
United Kingdom
phone: +44 (0)20 7479 7730
e-mail: info@dignityindying.org.uk • website: www.dignityindying.org.uk

Dignity in Dying believes that everyone has the right to a dignified death, and this means control over how one dies. It campaigns to change laws so that assisted death is legal for terminally ill, mentally competent adults who meet strict safeguards and feel their suffering has become unbearable. Its website contains information about assisted dying and many personal stories.

Division of Transplantation (DoT)
www.organdonor.gov

DoT is the federal entity responsible for overseeing the organ transplant system in the United States. Its website provides information about organ donation in the United States, including how the donation system works.

The Hastings Center
21 Malcolm Gordon Rd.
Garrison, NY 10524
phone: (845) 424-4040
website: www.thehastingscenter.org

The Hastings Center, founded in 1969, is a nonpartisan, nonprofit bioethics research institute. Its researchers address ethical issues in health, medicine, and the environment. Its website includes information about numerous bioethics topics.

Kennedy Institute of Ethics
Healy Hall, 4th Floor
Georgetown University
Washington, DC 20057
phone: (202) 687-8099
e-mail: kicourse@georgetown.edu • website: http://kennedyinstitute.ge orgetown.edu

The Kennedy Institute of Ethics at Georgetown University was established in 1971 and aims to promote discussion of bioethical issues. It publishes the *Kennedy Institute of Ethics Journal*, and its website has a large research library.

National Human Genome Research Institute
National Institutes of Health, Building 31, Room 4B09
31 Center Dr., MSC 2152
9000 Rockville Pike
Bethesda, MD 20892-2152
phone: (301) 402-0911 • fax: (301) 402-2218
website: www.genome.gov

The National Human Genome Research Institute began as the federal government's project to map the human genome. In addition, it works to apply genome technologies to the study of various diseases. Its website contains information about genetics and numerous ethical issues.

National Library of Medicine
8600 Rockville Pike
Bethesda, MD 20894
phone: (888) 346-3656 • fax: (301) 402-1384
website: www.nlm.nih.gov

The National Library of Medicine is the world's largest medical library. It provides information about all areas of biomedicine and health care.

For Further Research

Books

Donna Dickenson, *Bioethics*. London: Hodder Education, 2012.

Lee Gutkind and Pagan Kennedy, *An Immense New Power to Heal: The Promise of Personalized Medicine*. Pittsburgh, PA: In Fact, 2012.

Stephen Holland, ed., *Arguing About Bioethics*. New York: Routledge, 2012.

Muireabb Quigley, Sarah Chan, and John Harris, *Stem Cells: New Frontiers in Science & Ethics*. Singapore: World Scientific, 2012.

Marianne Talbot, *Bioethics: An Introduction*. New York: Cambridge University Press, 2012.

Periodicals

Daniel Allott and Neumary George, "Eugenic Abortion 2.0: A New Blood Test Could Zero Out the Disabled Unborn in the 21st Century," *American Spectator*, May 2013.

Tyler Cabot, "Whatever Happened to Stem Cells?," *Esquire*, April 2013.

Ethics Committee of the American Society for Reproductive Medicine, "Donating Embryos for Human Embryonic Stem Cell (hESC) Research: A Committee Opinion," *Fertility and Sterility*, October 2013.

Reed Karaim, "Assisted Suicide," *CQ Researcher*, May 17, 2013.

Daniella Lamas, "To Donate Your Kidney, Click Here," *New Yorker*, September 25, 2013.

José Pereira, "Legalizing Euthanasia or Assisted Suicide: The Illusion of Safeguards and Controls," *Current Oncology*, vol. 18, no. 2, 2011.

Paula Span, "Who Should Receive Organ Transplants?," *New York Times*, January 8, 2013.

Internet Sources

Howard Ball, Philip Nitschke, and Patrick Lee, "The Last Choice: Death and Dignity in the United States," *Cato Unbound*, December 2012. www.cato-unbound.org/issues/december-2012/last-choice-death-dignity-united-states.

National Human Genome Research Institute, "Issues in Genetics," November 1, 2013. www.genome.gov/Issues.

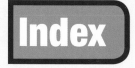

Index

Note: Boldface page numbers indicate illustrations.

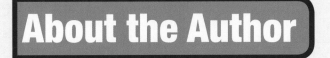

About the Author

Andrea C. Nakaya, a native of New Zealand, holds a BA in English and an MA in communications from San Diego State University. She has written and edited numerous books on current issues. She currently lives in Encinitas, California, with her husband and their two children, Natalie and Shane.